HEALTHY AGING AND NUTRITION FOR SENIORS

Nutritious Recipes for Seniors

BY MICHELLE HAUGER

TABEL OF CONTENTS

CONCLUSION

INTRODUCTION

As we progress through life, one of the most rewarding and fulfilling aspects is aging gracefully while maintaining our health and well-being. Healthy aging is a process that involves making conscious lifestyle choices and embracing nutritious habits to enhance the quality of life in our later years. For seniors, prioritizing proper nutrition becomes even more critical as it directly impacts their overall health, vitality, and longevity.

Nutrition plays a pivotal role in aging, influencing the body's resilience and ability to fight illnesses and chronic conditions. As we age, our bodies undergo various changes, including a decrease in metabolism, changes in taste and smell perception, and alterations in nutrient absorption. These factors make it crucial for seniors to follow a diet that caters to their specific nutritional needs.

A nutritious and well-balanced diet can help seniors maintain a healthy weight, promote bone health, regulate blood pressure and cholesterol levels, increase immunological function, and even lower the chance of acquiring age-related disorders such as heart disease, diabetes, and cognitive decline. Additionally, proper nutrition is essential for preserving muscle mass and strength, which are critical for maintaining mobility and independence as we age.

Preparing meals that are not only nutritious but also enjoyable is key to promoting healthy eating habits for seniors. While specific dietary requirements may vary from person to person, there are general guidelines that can serve as a foundation for crafting senior-friendly recipes.

Emphasizing whole foods is essential. Add fruits, vegetables, whole grains, lean proteins, and healthy fats into daily meals. Essential vitamins, minerals, and antioxidants included in these foods improve overall well-being. Additionally, as metabolism tends to slow down with age, attentive portion sizes should be taken into account.

Paying attention to portion control can help avoid overeating and maintain a healthy weight. Staying well-hydrated is also crucial for seniors, as aging can diminish the sensation of thirst. Encourage them to drink plenty of water, herbal teas, and natural juices. It's crucial to limit processed foods and sugar as they provide little nutritional value and can cause a variety of health problems. Put more emphasis on nutritious, nutrient-dense foods.

Adapting recipes for any dietary restrictions or medical conditions seniors may have is essential. Modifying recipes to meet their needs ensures they enjoy delicious meals without compromising their health.

In this guide, we will appropriately address the science of aging gracefully and explore a wealth of tasty and nutritious meals customized precisely to seniors' nutritional needs. Our mission is to provide a beneficial resource for elders and caregivers to help them make educated decisions, improve their well-being, and enjoy the journey of aging while embracing health and vitality. So let us go on this enlightening gastronomic journey that gracefully honors the art of aging!

SECTION ONE: KEY NUTRIENTS FOR ACTIVE SENIORS

Staying active becomes increasingly important as we age to maintain overall health and well-being. Numerous advantages come from regular physical activity, including better cardiovascular health, more flexibility, and more vitality.

For seniors who lead an active lifestyle, proper nutrition is vital to supporting their activity levels and overall vitality.

As active seniors strive to enjoy life fully, certain key nutrients support their unique needs. These nutrients provide essential sustenance and aid in promoting healthy aging, reducing the risk of chronic diseases, and supporting optimal physical function. Explore the essential vitamins, minerals, and other dietary components active seniors should prioritize.

Protein-Rich Recipes For Muscle Maintenance And Strength

For seniors to support their mobility, independence, and general wellbeing, it is essential to maintain muscular mass and strength. Muscle health and repair depend heavily on protein, a necessary nutrient. Incorporating protein-rich recipes into seniors' diets can help them stay active, strong, and healthy.

Here are protein-packed and delicious recipes for seniors to enhance their health and well-being:

1. Grilled Salmon with Quinoa and Roasted Vegetables

Ingredients:

- 2 salmon fillets

- 1 cup quinoa, cooked
- 1 cup mixed vegetables (e.g., bell peppers, zucchini, carrots)
- 2 tablespoons olive oil
- 1 tablespoon lemon juice
- 1 teaspoon of dry herbs, like rosemary or thyme. As desired, add salt and pepper.

Instructions:

1. Set the oven's temperature to 400°F (200°C). Combine the olive oil, dry herbs, salt, and pepper with the mixed veggies. They should be tender after 20 to 25 minutes in the oven.

2. Season the salmon fillets with lemon juice, salt, and pepper. Grill the salmon on each side for 4-5 minutes until cooked through. Place the grilled salmon on top of a delightful combination of cooked quinoa and roasted vegetables.

2. Greek Yogurt Parfait with Berries and Nuts

Ingredients:

- 1 cup Greek yogurt (low-fat or full-fat, as preferred)
- 1/2 cup mixed berries (blueberries, strawberries, raspberries)
- 2 tablespoons chopped nuts (almonds, walnuts, or pecans)
- 1 tablespoon honey or maple syrup (optional)

Instructions:

1. Layer Greek yogurt, mixed berries, and chopped nuts in a glass or bowl. For added sweetness, drizzle honey or maple syrup over the top, if desired.

3. Chickpea and Vegetable Stir-Fry

Ingredients:

- 1 can chickpeas, drained and rinsed
- 1 cup broccoli florets
- 1 red bell pepper, sliced
- 1 small onion, sliced
- 2 cloves garlic, minced
- 2 tablespoons of soy sauce (or, for a gluten-free alternative, tamari)
- 1 tablespoon sesame oil
- 1 tablespoon sesame seeds
- Cooked brown rice or quinoa for serving

Instructions:

1. Over medium heat, heat the sesame oil in a big skillet.

2. Sauté minced garlic for a minute, then add sliced onions, bell peppers, and broccoli florets to the skillet. Stir-fry the vegetables for 5-6 minutes until they reach a tender-crisp consistency.

3. Toss in the chickpeas and soy sauce, combining everything well in the skillet. Lastly, sprinkle sesame seeds over the stir-fry and serve it atop cooked brown rice or quinoa.

4. Turkey and Vegetable Wrap

Ingredients:

- 4 whole-grain tortillas or wraps
- 8 slices of roasted turkey (or any lean protein of choice)
- 1 cup baby spinach leaves
- 1/2 cup sliced cucumber

- 1/2 cup shredded carrots
- 2 tablespoons hummus or Greek yogurt dressing (as a spread)

Instructions:

1. Place the tortillas on a flat surface and spread a thin layer of hummus or Greek yogurt dressing on each of them. Place two slices of roasted turkey on each tortilla, followed by baby spinach, sliced cucumber, and shredded carrots.

2. Roll up the tortillas tightly to form wraps. Cut them in half and serve as a satisfying lunch or a light dinner option rich in protein.

5. Lentil and Vegetable Soup

Ingredients:

- 1 cup dried green or red lentils
- 1 large carrot, diced
- 1 celery stalk, diced
- 1 small onion, chopped
- 2 cloves garlic, minced
- 1 can diced tomatoes
- 4 cups vegetable or chicken broth
- 1 teaspoon ground cumin
- 1/2 teaspoon ground coriander
- Salt and pepper to taste
- Fresh parsley for garnish

Instructions:

1. Sauté the chopped onions, garlic, diced carrots, and celery in a large pot until they soften. Add the lentils, diced tomatoes, ground cumin, ground coriander, salt,

and pepper to the pot. Stir everything together to combine.

2. Bring the soup to a boil while adding the chicken or veggie broth. Lower the heat to a simmer until it starts to boil, and then cover the pot. Allow it to simmer for 20 to 25 minutes, or until the lentils have become tender.

These protein-rich recipes provide essential nutrients to support muscle maintenance and strength in seniors. Along with regular physical activity, incorporating these delicious and nutritious meals into their diets will help seniors lead active and vibrant lives while promoting their overall health and well-being.

High-Protein Breakfast Recipes to Kickstart the Day

Incorporate these nutrient-packed meals into your morning routine to fuel your body, stay full longer, and set the tone for a productive day.

1. Spinach and Feta Omelette

Ingredients:

- 3 large eggs
- 1 cup fresh spinach, chopped
- 1/4 cup crumbled feta cheese
- 1/4 cup diced tomatoes
- 1/4 cup diced bell peppers
- 1 tablespoon olive oil
- Salt and pepper to taste

Instructions:

1. Add salt and pepper to the eggs after whisking them in a bowl. In a nonstick skillet over medium heat, warm up the olive oil. Add the chopped spinach to the tomatoes and bell peppers after they have cooked through.

2. Pour the whisked eggs into the skillet, spreading them evenly. Sprinkle crumbled feta cheese over the eggs.

3. Cook the omelet for 2-3 minutes until the edges are set. Then, fold it in half and cook for another minute to ensure it's fully cooked.

2. Quinoa Breakfast Bowl

Ingredients:

- 1 cup cooked quinoa
- 1/2 cup plain Greek yogurt
- 1/4 cup fresh berries (blueberries, raspberries, strawberries)
- 2 tablespoons chopped almonds or walnuts
- 1 tablespoon honey or maple syrup (optional)

Instructions:

1. For added crunch and protein, sprinkle chopped nuts on top. If you prefer sweetness, drizzle honey or maple syrup over the bowl.

2. Mix all the ingredients to create a delightful and protein-rich breakfast option.

3. High-Protein Smoothie Bowl

Ingredients:

- 1 ripe banana

- 1/2 cup frozen mixed berries (blueberries, raspberries, strawberries)
- 1/2 cup plain Greek yogurt
- 1/4 cup milk (dairy or plant-based)
- 1 tablespoon almond butter or peanut butter
- 1 tablespoon chia seeds
- Toppings: sliced fruits, granola, shredded coconut, and a drizzle of honey

Instructions:

1. Combine the banana, frozen berries, Greek yogurt, milk, almond butter, and chia seeds in a blender. Blend the ingredients until smooth and creamy, adjusting the milk amount to achieve your desired consistency.

2. Pour the smoothie into a bowl and arrange your favorite toppings as desired.

4. Egg and Avocado Toast

Ingredients:

- 2 slices whole-grain bread, toasted
- 2 large eggs
- 1 ripe avocado, mashed
- 1 teaspoon lemon juice
- Salt and pepper to taste
- Red pepper flakes (optional for added spice)

Instructions:

1. Start by mashing the avocado in a small bowl with lemon juice, salt, and pepper. Poach or fry the eggs according to your preference. Evenly spread the mashed avocado on toasted bread slices.

2. Place a poached or fried egg on top of each slice.
   Sprinkle some red pepper flakes if desired for an extra
   kick.

5. Cottage Cheese and Fruit Parfait

Ingredients:

- 1 cup low-fat cottage cheese
- 1/2 cup mixed fresh fruits (pineapple, kiwi, mango, or any favorites)
- 2 tablespoons granola
- 1 tablespoon honey

Instructions:

1. Layer the cottage cheese and mixed fresh fruits in a glass or bowl. Add a sprinkle of granola on top for some crunch and texture.

2. Drizzle honey over the parfait to add natural sweetness and mix all the layers together to combine the flavors and textures.

These high-protein breakfast recipes are delicious and provide the energy and nourishment needed to kickstart the day on a positive note.

Protein-Packed Recipes For Sustained Energy

Protein is a vital nutrient crucial in providing sustained energy, supporting muscle maintenance, and promoting overall well-being. These protein-packed recipes are designed to energize you throughout the day and enhance your strength and vitality.

1. Buttery Shrimp with Marinated White Beans

Ingredients:

- 1 lb large shrimp, peeled and deveined
- 2 tablespoons unsalted butter
- 2 cloves garlic, minced
- 1 teaspoon paprika
- 1/2 teaspoon dried thyme
- Salt and pepper to taste
- 2 cans white beans (cannellini beans), drained and rinsed
- 1/4 cup extra-virgin olive oil
- 2 tablespoons lemon juice
- 1 tablespoon chopped fresh parsley
- Lemon wedges for serving

Instructions:

Marinating the White Beans:

1. Mix the drained and rinsed white beans in a medium-sized bowl with extra-virgin olive oil and lemon juice.

2. Add chopped fresh parsley, salt, and pepper to the beans. Thoroughly combine all the ingredients, ensuring the beans are evenly coated with the marinade. Set the marinated white beans aside to let the flavors meld.

Preparing the Buttery Shrimp:

1. Melt the unsalted butter in a large skillet over medium heat. Sauté the minced garlic in the melted butter until it becomes fragrant.

2. Next, add the peeled and deveined shrimp to the skillet. Sprinkle paprika, dried thyme, salt, and pepper over the

shrimp. Cook the shrimp on each side for 2-3 minutes until they turn pink and are thoroughly cooked. Finally, take the skillet off the heat.

Serving the Buttery Shrimp with Marinated White Beans:

1. Start by arranging the marinated white beans on a serving platter. Place the buttery shrimp on top of the white beans for an enticing combination.

2. Garnish the dish with additional chopped fresh parsley for a pop of color and freshness. For an extra burst of citrusy flavor, serve the flavorful, buttery shrimp with marinated white beans and lemon wedges.

2.- Peanut Butter Banana Smoothie

Ingredients:

- 1 ripe banana
- 2 tablespoons natural peanut butter
- 1 cup Greek yogurt (low-fat or full-fat, as preferred)
- 1/2 cup milk (dairy or plant-based)
- 1 tablespoon honey (optional for added sweetness)
- Ice cubes (optional)

Instructions:

Combine the ripe banana, peanut butter, Greek yogurt, and milk in a blender. You may include honey in the mixture if you'd like it even sweeter.

1. For a thicker and cooler smoothie, toss in some ice cubes. Blend all the ingredients until the smoothie becomes smooth and creamy. Then, pour the smoothie

into a glass and savor the delightful flavors of this nutritious peanut butter banana smoothie.

3. One-Pot Italian Sausage-Gnocchi Soup

Ingredients:

- 1 lb Italian sausage, casings removed
- 1 onion, diced
- 3 cloves garlic, minced
- 4 cups chicken broth
- 1 can (14.5 oz) diced tomatoes
- 1 cup tomato sauce
- 1 teaspoon dried basil
- 1 teaspoon dried oregano
- 1/2 teaspoon red pepper flakes (optional for added spice)
- 1 package (16 oz) potato gnocchi
- 2 cups fresh spinach
- Salt and pepper to taste
- Grated Parmesan cheese for garnish
- Fresh basil leaves for garnish (optional)

Instructions:

1. Get a large pot or Dutch oven. Heat it over medium heat, and add the Italian sausage. As it cooks, break it into crumbles using a spatula or spoon. Toss in the diced onions and sauté them until they turn translucent. Once that's done, stir in the minced garlic and cook for about a minute until you can smell its fragrant aroma.

2. Pour in the chicken broth, diced tomatoes, and tomato sauce. If you like a bit of heat, stir in some dried basil, dried oregano, and red pepper flakes. Bring the soup to a boil and lower the heat to a simmer. Cover the pot and

let it cook for approximately 10 minutes so the flavors can meld together.

3. While the soup simmers, add the potato gnocchi to the pot. Follow the package instructions to cook them, which usually takes 2-3 minutes. Once the gnocchi is perfectly cooked, toss in the fresh spinach. Stir until the spinach wilts and blends nicely into the soup. Now, season the soup with salt and pepper according to your preference.

4. To serve, ladle the delicious Italian Sausage-Gnocchi Soup into bowls. You can garnish each serving with grated Parmesan cheese and fresh basil leaves if you like.

4. Turkey-Pumpkin Chili

Ingredients:

- 1 lb ground turkey
- 1 onion, diced
- 3 cloves garlic, minced
- 1 can (15 oz) pumpkin puree
- 1 can (15 oz) black beans, drained and rinsed
- 1 can (15 oz) kidney beans, drained and rinsed
- 1 can (14.5 oz) diced tomatoes
- 2 cups chicken or vegetable broth
- 2 tablespoons chili powder
- 1 teaspoon cumin
- 1/2 teaspoon cinnamon
- Salt and pepper to taste
- Olive oil for cooking
- Shredded cheddar cheese and chopped green onions for garnish

Instructions:

1. Start by heating a drizzle of olive oil over medium heat in a pot. Add diced onions and sauté until they become translucent. Stir in minced garlic and cook for another minute until it becomes fragrant. Add ground turkey to the pot and cook until it is browned, breaking it into crumbles as it cooks. Pour in pumpkin puree, black beans, kidney beans, diced tomatoes, and chicken or vegetable broth.

2. Season the chili with chili powder, cumin, cinnamon, salt, and pepper. Bring the chili to a simmer and let it cook for about 20-25 minutes, stirring occasionally. Once the Turkey-Pumpkin Chili is ready, serve it in bowls and garnish each serving with shredded cheddar cheese and chopped green onions.

5. Roasted Root Veggie Quinoa Bowls

Ingredients:

- 1 cup quinoa, rinsed and drained
- 2 cups vegetable broth or water
- 2 cups mixed root vegetables (carrots, sweet potatoes, beets, parsnips), peeled and diced
- 2 tablespoons olive oil
- 1 teaspoon dried thyme
- Salt and pepper to taste
- 2 cups baby spinach or mixed greens
- 1/4 cup crumbled feta cheese or goat cheese (optional)
- Balsamic vinaigrette dressing for drizzling (optional)

Instructions:

1. Preheat the oven until it's hot. In a saucepan, bring vegetable broth or water to a boil. Add quinoa, then lower the heat, cover, and let it simmer for around 15

minutes or until the quinoa is cooked and fluffy. Prepare diced root vegetables with olive oil, dried thyme, salt, and pepper.

2. Spread the seasoned vegetables on a baking sheet and roast in the oven until tender and slightly caramelized, usually taking about 20-25 minutes. Layer cooked quinoa, roasted root vegetables, and baby spinach or mixed greens in individual serving bowls. If desired, sprinkle crumbled feta or goat cheese over the bowls. For added flavor, drizzle with balsamic vinaigrette dressing.

These delicious and wholesome recipes are packed with protein and provide a comforting and nutritious meal for any occasion. From hearty soups to flavorful chili and nourishing quinoa bowls, these dishes will keep you energized and satisfied while promoting overall health and well-being.

Nourishing Dinner Recipes to Support Muscle Health

These nourishing dinner recipes have been thoughtfully curated to provide essential nutrients and protein, supporting muscle maintenance and strength in seniors.

1. Air Fryer Turkey Burgers

Ingredients:

- 1 lb ground turkey
- 1/4 cup breadcrumbs
- 1/4 cup diced onion
- 1/4 cup chopped parsley
- 1 teaspoon garlic powder
- 1 teaspoon onion powder
- 1/2 teaspoon salt
- 1/4 teaspoon black pepper

- 4 whole wheat burger buns
- Lettuce, tomato slices, and other toppings of your choice
- Condiments (ketchup, mustard, mayonnaise) as desired

Instructions:

1. In a mixing bowl, combine ground turkey, breadcrumbs, diced onion, chopped parsley, garlic powder, onion powder, salt, and black pepper. Thoroughly mix everything together until well combined.

2. Shape the mixture into four burger patties. Preheat your air fryer until it reaches 375°F (190°C). To ensure equal cooking, turn the turkey burger patties halfway through cooking. Place the turkey burger patties in the air fryer basket and cook for 10 to 12 minutes.

3. Once the burgers are fully cooked and have reached a safe internal temperature, assemble them on whole wheat burger buns, and add your favorite toppings and condiments.

2. Italian-Inspired Beef & Farro Bowls

Ingredients:

- 1 lb ground beef
- 1 cup farro, cooked according to package instructions
- 1 cup cherry tomatoes, halved
- 1/2 cup chopped cucumber
- 1/4 cup sliced black olives
- 1/4 cup crumbled feta cheese
- 2 tablespoons balsamic vinegar
- 2 tablespoons extra-virgin olive oil
- 1 teaspoon dried oregano

- Salt and pepper to taste

Instructions:

1. Start by cooking the ground beef in a skillet over medium heat until it is browned and fully cooked. Make sure to drain any excess fat. Combine cooked farro, cherry tomatoes, chopped cucumber, sliced black olives, and crumbled feta cheese in a large bowl.

2. In a separate small bowl, whisk together balsamic vinegar, extra-virgin olive oil, dried oregano, salt, and pepper to create the dressing. Add the cooked ground beef to the farro and vegetable mixture, and toss everything with the dressing until it is well coated.

3. Creamy Polenta Shrimp and Vegetable Bowls

Ingredients:

- 1 cup polenta (cornmeal)
- 4 cups vegetable or chicken broth
- 1 lb large shrimp, peeled and deveined
- 1 cup chopped broccoli florets
- 1 cup sliced bell peppers (mixed colors)
- 1/2 cup sliced cherry tomatoes
- 1/4 cup grated Parmesan cheese
- 2 tablespoons olive oil
- 2 cloves garlic, minced
- 1 tablespoon chopped fresh parsley
- Salt and pepper to taste

Instructions:

1. In a saucepan, bring vegetable or chicken broth to a boil. Slowly whisk in the polenta and then reduce the heat to low. Continue to cook the polenta, stirring

frequently, until it thickens and becomes creamy, usually taking around 20 minutes.

2. Meanwhile, in a large skillet, heat olive oil over medium-high heat. Sauté minced garlic for about a minute. Add shrimp to the skillet until they turn pink and are cooked through. Once cooked, remove the shrimp from the skillet and set them aside.

3. In the same skillet, sauté chopped broccoli florets and sliced bell peppers until they reach a tender-crisp texture. Stir in sliced cherry tomatoes and the cooked shrimp. Season the shrimp and vegetable mixture with salt and pepper to taste.

4. Serve the creamy polenta in bowls, and top it with the flavorful shrimp and vegetable mixture. For added flavor and presentation, sprinkle grated Parmesan cheese and chopped fresh parsley over the dish. Enjoy this delightful and satisfying meal!

4. Vegan Fried Tofu Sandwich

Ingredients:

- 1 block of firm tofu, sliced into 1/2-inch thick pieces
- 1/2 cup all-purpose flour
- 1/2 cup plant-based milk (almond, soy, or any preferred)
- 1 cup breadcrumbs (panko or regular)
- 1 teaspoon paprika
- 1/2 teaspoon garlic powder
- 1/4 teaspoon salt
- 1/4 teaspoon black pepper
- Olive oil for frying
- Whole grain bread slices

- Lettuce, tomato slices, avocado slices, and other toppings of your choice
- Vegan mayo or mustard for spreading

Instructions:

1. Prepare a dredging station by setting up three shallow bowls. Place all-purpose flour in one bowl, pour plant-based milk into the second bowl, and combine breadcrumbs, paprika, garlic powder, salt, and black pepper in the third bowl.

2. Dip each tofu slice into the flour first, then the plant-based milk, and finally, coat it with the breadcrumb mixture, gently pressing to ensure the coating adheres.

3. In a skillet, heat olive oil over medium-high heat. Add the breaded tofu slices and cook until they become golden brown and crispy on both sides.

4. Once the fried tofu slices are ready, remove them from the skillet and place them on a plate lined with paper towels to absorb any excess oil. Spread vegan mayo or mustard on slices of whole-grain bread.

5. Assemble the vegan fried tofu sandwich by layering lettuce, tomato slices, avocado slices, and crispy tofu.

5. Baked Bean Pizza

Ingredients:

- 1 pre-made pizza dough or homemade pizza dough
- 1 cup canned baked beans
- 1/2 cup shredded mozzarella cheese
- 1/2 cup diced cooked ham or bacon (optional)
- 1/4 cup diced red onion
- 1/4 cup diced bell peppers (mixed colors)

- 1 tablespoon olive oil
- 1 teaspoon dried oregano
- Fresh parsley for garnish (optional)

Instructions:

1. Preheat your oven to the temperature specified in the pizza dough instructions or to 425°F (220°C) if you use homemade dough.

2. Roll out the pizza dough to your desired thickness on a floured surface. Transfer the pizza dough to a baking sheet or pizza stone. Evenly spread the canned baked beans on the pizza dough, leaving a border around the edges. Sprinkle shredded mozzarella cheese over the beans.

3. If you are using diced cooked ham or bacon, add it next, followed by diced red onion and bell peppers. Then, drizzle olive oil over the pizza toppings.

4. Now, bake the pizza in the oven until the crust is golden brown and the cheese has melted and bubbled. This should take approximately 12-15 minutes, but the timing may vary depending on your oven and dough thickness.

5. Once the pizza is cooked to your satisfaction, take it out of the oven, let it cool for a moment, then slice and enjoy your delicious homemade baked bean pizza!

SECTION TWO: HEART-HEALTH

The heart, a tireless organ, is at the core of our well-being, tirelessly pumping life into every cell of our body. Caring for heart health is crucial for a vibrant and fulfilling life. Heart health encompasses a range of lifestyle choices, dietary habits, and physical activities that work harmoniously to support this essential lifeline's strength and vitality.

Taking care of our hearts is crucial in preventing heart disease, and it requires a continuous commitment to nourishing our bodies and minds. Through mindful decisions in our daily routines, we can support our hearts and enhance their well-being, leading to a longer and healthier life while lowering the likelihood of cardiovascular problems.

Heart-Healthy Recipes For Cardiovascular Health

The foundation of our overall well-being lies in having a healthy heart, and one of the key factors in promoting cardiovascular health is making conscious decisions about the food we eat. These heart-healthy recipes are designed to provide nourishment and strengthen our hearts. The risk of heart disease, high blood pressure, and cholesterol levels can be significantly decreased by adopting a diet rich in minerals, antioxidants, and healthy fats. Let's enjoy these delectable dishes to encourage a robust and forgiving heart.

1. Beet and Carrot Salad with Ginger

Ingredients:

- 2 large beets, peeled and grated
- 2 large carrots, peeled and grated
- 1-inch piece of fresh ginger, grated

- 2 tablespoons lemon juice
- 2 tablespoons extra-virgin olive oil
- 1 tablespoon honey or maple syrup.
- Salt and pepper to taste
- Fresh parsley or cilantro for garnish

Instructions:

1. Grate the carrots and beets, then place them in a big basin. The dressing is made by blending extra virgin olive oil, grated ginger, lemon juice, and, if preferred, honey or maple syrup in a separate small bowl.

2. Make sure all of the beet and carrot components are well-coated by thoroughly tossing the mixture with the dressing. Your taste for salt and pepper should be used to season the salad.

3. Add fresh parsley or cilantro as a garnish before serving to give the salad a flavorful and eye-catching boost. This tasty side dish or light lunch alternative is this heart-healthy, reviving beet and carrot salad.

2. Tangy Tomato Soup with Basil

Ingredients:

- 1 tablespoon olive oil
- 1 large onion, chopped
- 3 cloves garlic, minced
- 28 ounces canned crushed tomatoes
- 4 cups vegetable broth
- 1 tablespoon balsamic vinegar
- 1 teaspoon dried basil
- Salt and pepper to taste
- Fresh basil leaves for garnish

Instructions:

1. Start by bringing olive oil to a simmer in a big saucepan over medium heat. The chopped onions should be cooked until they become transparent. When the air is fragrant, add the minced garlic and simmer for one more minute.

2. Then add the vegetable broth, balsamic vinegar, dried basil, salt, and pepper to the saucepan along with the smashed tomatoes in a can. The soup should be brought to a mild boil before being simmered. For 15 to 20 minutes, cover the saucepan and mix the ingredients regularly to achieve equal cooking.

3. After the flavors have harmoniously combined, mix the soup with an immersion blender until it is utterly smooth.

4. Finally, serve this tangy tomato soup with a garnish of fresh basil leaves, not only for added flavor but also to elevate its presentation. Embrace this tomato soup's heart-healthy and comforting goodness, perfect as a satisfying appetizer or light and wholesome dinner option.

3. Barley Soup with Beans and Basil

Ingredients:

- 1 cup pearl barley
- 4 cups vegetable broth
- 1 can (15 ounces) kidney beans, drained and rinsed
- One can (15 ounces) chickpeas, drained and rinsed
- 1 cup diced tomatoes
- 1 cup chopped carrots
- 1 cup chopped celery
- 1 large onion, chopped

- 3 cloves garlic, minced
- 1 tablespoon olive oil
- 1 teaspoon dried basil
- Salt and pepper to taste
- Fresh basil leaves for garnish

Instructions:

1. On medium heat, first, warm up the olive oil in a big saucepan. The minced garlic should be added after the chopped onions have become translucent and have given off a lovely aroma, about one more minute.

2. Subsequently, add the chopped carrots and celery to the saucepan and stir-fry them for a few minutes or until they begin to soften.

3. Bring it to a boil after adding the veggie broth. Add salt, pepper, dried basil, chopped tomatoes, kidney beans, chickpeas, pearl barley, and chickpeas to the saucepan. Simmer the soup by reducing the heat, covering the pot, and letting it cook for 30 to 40 minutes until the barley and vegetables are tender.

4. Before serving, garnish this comforting barley soup with fresh basil leaves to add a touch of brightness and flavor. Savor the wholesome goodness of this nourishing soup!

4. Super-Nutritious Broccoli Salad with Apples and Cranberries

Ingredients:

- 4 cups broccoli florets
- 1 large apple, diced
- 1/2 cup dried cranberries
- 1/2 cup chopped walnuts or almonds

- 1/4 cup diced red onion
- 1/4 cup plain Greek yogurt
- 2 tablespoons apple cider vinegar
- 1 tablespoon honey or maple syrup
- Salt and pepper to taste

Instructions:

1. Combine broccoli florets, diced apple, dried cranberries, chopped walnuts or almonds, and diced red onion in a large mixing dish.

2. To prepare the dressing, combine the plain Greek yogurt, apple cider vinegar, honey or maple syrup, salt and pepper in a separate bowl.

3. When the ingredients are thoroughly coated, pour the dressing over the broccoli salad and stir to combine. If necessary, add extra salt and pepper after tasting the salad. To enhance the flavors, it's recommended to refrigerate the salad for at least thirty minutes before serving, giving the ingredients time to blend harmoniously. Savor the delightful and hydrating taste of this broccoli salad!

5. Grilled Salmon with Citrus Salsa

Ingredients:

- 4 salmon fillets (about 6 ounces each)
- 2 tablespoons olive oil
- 1 teaspoon smoked paprika
- Salt and pepper to taste

Citrus Salsa:

- 1 orange, peeled and diced
- 1 grapefruit, peeled and diced

- 1 small red onion, finely chopped
- 1 tablespoon fresh lime juice
- 2 tablespoons chopped fresh cilantro
- Salt and pepper to taste

Instructions:

1. Begin preparing the grilled salmon by preheating the grill to medium-high heat. Brush olive oil over the salmon fillets and generously sprinkle them with smoked paprika, salt, and pepper. Grill the seasoned salmon for 4-5 minutes on each side or until it becomes easily flaky when tested with a fork.

2. In a bowl, mix diced orange, grapefruit, red onion, lime juice, and chopped cilantro to create a vibrant citrus salsa. Season the salsa with salt and pepper according to your taste preferences.

3. Serve the grilled salmon with a generous spoonful of the refreshing citrus salsa to infuse the dish with fresh and invigorating flavors. Enjoy this delectable and healthy meal!

6. Baked Herb-Crusted Chicken

Ingredients:

- 4 boneless, skinless chicken breasts
- 1/2 cup whole wheat breadcrumbs
- 2 tablespoons grated Parmesan cheese
- 1 teaspoon dried thyme
- 1 teaspoon dried rosemary
- 1/2 teaspoon garlic powder
- 1/2 teaspoon onion powder
- Salt and pepper to taste
- 2 tablespoons olive oil

Instructions:

1. Preheat your oven as directed. In a shallow dish, combine whole wheat breadcrumbs, grated Parmesan cheese, rosemary, dried thyme, garlic powder, onion powder, salt, and pepper.

2. Coat each chicken breast with a brush of olive oil, followed by dipping them into the breadcrumb mixture, gently pressing to ensure the coating sticks. Place the herb-crusted chicken breasts onto a baking sheet in preparation for cooking.

3. Allow the chicken to bake in the oven for approximately 25-30 minutes or until it is thoroughly cooked and the crust has a delightful golden and crispy appearance. Relish this scrumptious and nutritious meal!

7. Berry Spinach Salad with Walnuts

Ingredients:

- 4 cups baby spinach
- 1 cup mixed berries (blueberries, raspberries, strawberries)
- 1/4 one-fourth cup of crumbled goat cheese or feta cheese
- 1/4 cup chopped walnuts
- 2 tablespoons balsamic vinaigrette dressing (or dressing of your choice)

Instructions:

1. Place baby spinach, mixed berries, crumbled goat cheese or feta cheese, and chopped walnuts in a large salad bowl. Drizzle the balsamic vinaigrette dressing over the ingredients and toss everything together until

thoroughly combined. Enjoy this delicious and refreshing salad!

2. These heart-healthy recipes are delicious and satisfying and play a significant role in preventing cardiovascular problems. These recipes promote heart health, maintain a healthy weight, and support overall well-being by incorporating nutrient-rich ingredients and wholesome components like salmon, quinoa, beans, chickpeas, chicken, and fresh fruits and vegetables.

Delicious Dishes To Lower Cholesterol Levels

The risk of cholesterol-related issues increases as we become older. High cholesterol levels can cause cardiovascular difficulties, affecting the health and function of the heart. We can take proactive actions toward keeping a strong and resilient heart as we age by integrating cholesterol-lowering foods and heart-healthy ingredients into our diets.

Embracing a heart-healthy diet is vital to promoting overall well-being and supporting healthy aging. These recipes are not only delicious but also significantly reduce cholesterol levels and nourish the body as we age gracefully.

1. Chicken & Cucumber Lettuce Wraps with Peanut Sauce

Ingredients:

- One lb boneless, skinless chicken breast, cooked and shredded
- 1 cucumber, julienned
- 1 carrot, julienned
- 1/4 cup chopped fresh cilantro
- 1/4 cup chopped peanuts
- 8 large lettuce leaves (butter lettuce or romaine)

- Lime wedges for garnish
- Peanut Sauce:
- 1/4 cup creamy peanut butter
- One tablespoon of soy sauce (or tamari for gluten-free)
- 2 tablespoons honey or maple syrup
- 1 tablespoon rice vinegar
- 1 teaspoon sesame oil
- 1/2 teaspoon grated fresh ginger
- 1 clove garlic, minced
- 2-3 tablespoons water (to reach desired consistency)

Instructions:

1. Prepare the peanut sauce by whisking all the ingredients in a small bowl until you achieve a smooth consistency. Adjust the thickness with water as required.

2. Toss the cooked and shredded chicken, julienned cucumber, julienned carrot, chopped cilantro, and chopped peanuts together in a large mixing bowl until well combined.

3. Arrange the lettuce leaves on a clean surface. Spoon the chicken and vegetable mixture onto each lettuce leaf. Generously drizzle peanut sauce over the filling in each lettuce leaf. Relish the delightful and flavorful lettuce wraps!

4. Roll up the lettuce wraps and use toothpicks to secure them if needed. Enjoy this delicious and convenient meal!

5. Serve the chicken & cucumber lettuce wraps with peanut sauce as a delicious and cholesterol-friendly appetizer or light main course. Garnish with lime wedges for an extra burst of flavor.

These refreshing and nutrient-packed lettuce wraps are perfect for seniors looking to enjoy a satisfying and heart-healthy meal that supports their overall well-being and helps maintain cholesterol levels.

2. Seared Tuna with Bulgur & Chickpea Salad

Ingredients:

- 2 tuna steaks (about 6 ounces each)
- 1 cup cooked bulgur
- One can (15 ounces) chickpeas, drained and rinsed
- 1 cup cherry tomatoes, halved
- 1/2 cucumber, diced
- 1/4 cup chopped red onion
- 1/4 cup chopped fresh parsley
- 2 tablespoons lemon juice
- 2 tablespoons extra-virgin olive oil
- Salt and pepper to taste

Instructions:

1. Start by coating the tuna steaks on both sides with salt and pepper. Olive oil is added to a skillet or grill pan heated over medium-high heat. Depending on how you want your tuna steaks, grill them for 2 to 3 minutes on each side for the best flavor and texture. Save the tuna steaks once you're finished.

2. Mix the cooked bulgur, chickpeas, cherry tomatoes, sliced cucumber, red onion, and fresh parsley in a large bowl.

3. Using a separate bowl, mix the lemon juice properly, extra virgin olive oil, salt, and pepper to make the dressing.

4. Drizzle the dressing over the bulgur and chickpea salad, and toss everything together until thoroughly combined. Enjoy this flavorful and nutritious salad!

5. Serve the flavorful tuna steaks alongside the refreshing bulgur and chickpea salad. Enjoy this delicious and nutritious meal!

3. Sweet Potato-Black Bean Burgers

Ingredients:

- 2 cups cooked sweet potatoes, mashed
- One Can of black beans,
- 1/2 cup cooked quinoa
- 1/4 cup chopped fresh cilantro
- 1/4 cup chopped red onion
- 1 teaspoon ground cumin
- 1/2 teaspoon chili powder
- Salt and pepper to taste
- Whole grain burger buns
- Lettuce, tomato slices, avocado slices, and other toppings of your choice
- Olive oil for cooking

Instructions:

1. Using a large mixing bowl, mashed sweet potatoes, black beans, cooked quinoa, chopped cilantro, chopped red onion, ground cumin, chili powder, salt, and pepper. Mix everything thoroughly using a fork or potato masher until well combined.

2. Create burger patties from the sweet potato and black bean mixture. The sweet potato-black bean burgers should be cooked for 3 to 4 minutes on each side until golden and crispy. Remember to heat the olive oil in a pan over medium-high heat.

3. Assemble the sweet potato-black bean burgers on whole grain burger buns, topped with lettuce, tomato, avocado, and any other toppings of your choice. Enjoy these delectable and hearty burgers!

4. Pan-Seared Steak with Crispy Herbs & Escarole

Ingredients:

- 2 boneless beef steaks (about 8 ounces each)
- 2 tablespoons olive oil
- 3 cloves garlic, thinly sliced
- 1 tablespoon chopped fresh rosemary
- 1 tablespoon chopped fresh thyme
- Salt and pepper to taste
- 1 small head escarole, washed and chopped
- 1 tablespoon balsamic vinegar

Instructions:

1. The first step is to thoroughly coat the steaks in oil and season both sides with salt and pepper.

2. The steaks should now be carefully placed into a hot skillet or grill pan once the skillet or pan has been preheated over medium-high heat. To cook them to medium-rare doneness, allow them to cook for 3–4 minutes on each side, modifying the cooking time to your preference. The steaks should be removed from the skillet after they finish cooking and let to rest.

3. Thinly sliced garlic, fresh rosemary, and fresh thyme are cooked in the same skillet with more olive oil as necessary until the herbs are crisp. Discard the crispy herb mixture.

4. Next, sauté the chopped escarole in the same skillet until it wilts and becomes tender. Drizzle the escarole with balsamic vinegar and toss until it is well coated.

This flavorful and nutritious dish supports heart health and overall well-being, making it an excellent choice for seniors looking to enjoy a delicious and nourishing meal.

5. Instant Pot Chicken Soup with Root Vegetables & Barley

Ingredients:

- One lb of boneless, skinless chicken breasts or thighs
- 1 cup chopped carrots
- 1 cup chopped celery
- 1 cup chopped parsnips
- 1 cup chopped turnips
- 1/2 cup pearl barley
- 6 cups chicken broth
- 2 cloves garlic, minced
- 1 teaspoon dried thyme
- Salt and pepper to taste
- Fresh parsley for garnish (optional)

Instructions:

1. In the Instant Pot, combine chicken breasts or thighs, chopped carrots, chopped celery, chopped parsnips, chopped turnips, pearl barley, chicken broth, minced garlic, dried thyme, salt, and pepper. Set the valve to the sealing position and close the Instant Pot lid.

Depending on the thickness of the chicken, set the cooking time for 20 to 25 minutes under high pressure.

2. After the cooking process has finished, wait 5 minutes for a natural release before performing a fast release to let off any leftover pressure. Carefully remove the cooked chicken breasts or thighs from the Instant Pot by opening the lid.

3. With two forks, shred the chicken, then put it back in the pressure cooker. Stir the soup to thoroughly combine all the ingredients.

6. American Goulash

Ingredients:

- 1 lb ground beef or turkey
- 1 large onion, chopped
- 3 cloves garlic, minced
- 1 can (28 ounces) crushed tomatoes
- 2 cups beef or vegetable broth
- 2 cups elbow macaroni (whole wheat for a healthier option)
- 1 tablespoon olive oil
- 1 teaspoon paprika
- 1/2 teaspoon dried oregano
- 1/2 teaspoon dried basil
- Salt and pepper to taste
- Fresh parsley for garnish

Instructions:

1. Start by bringing olive oil to a medium-high heat in a large pan. When the onions are translucent, add them to the skillet and continue cooking them. Stir in the minced garlic when the garlic fragrance has filled the

air, and simmer for another minute. The ground beef or turkey should be cooked in the skillet until it is well-cooked and well-browned. Ensure that any excess fat is removed from the skillet.

2. Then add beef or vegetable broth, salt, pepper, paprika, dried oregano, dried basil, and smashed tomatoes to the pan. The components are combined by stirring. The mixture should be brought to a mild boil, then simmered for 15 to 20 minutes.

3. Cook the elbow macaroni until it is al dente in the meanwhile, following the directions on the package. The macaroni must be drained after cooking.

4. Add the cooked macaroni to the skillet with the beef and tomato mixture. Stir everything together until well combined. Enjoy this comforting and delicious meal!

These recipes are carefully crafted to lower cholesterol levels and promote cardiovascular health and well-being.

SECTION THREE: BONE-STRENGTHENING RECIPES

Our bones' strength and integrity form the foundation of our physical vitality. Maintaining strong and healthy bones becomes crucial to overall well-being as we age, particularly for seniors. The concern for bone health becomes even more pressing as the risk of conditions like osteoporosis looms closer.

Bone strengthening is a proactive approach to safeguarding the skeletal system, ensuring that bones remain resilient and can easily support our daily activities. A combination of factors, including a nutrient-rich diet, regular exercise, and lifestyle choices, significantly optimize bone health.

When aiming to strengthen our bones, nutrition plays a crucial role. It is essential to incorporate foods abundant in vital nutrients like calcium, vitamin D, magnesium, and phosphorus, as they significantly contribute to bone density and overall strength. Equally important is incorporating weight-bearing exercises that stimulate bone growth and maintenance.

This journey towards bone strengthening is not just about preventing fractures but promoting a life of vitality and independence. Seniors, in particular, can benefit immensely from adopting bone-strengthening practices, empowering them to age gracefully and maintain their mobility and agility.

Bone-Strengthening Recipes For Osteoporosis Prevention

The bone-strengthening recipes have been meticulously designed to provide vital vitamins and minerals that promote strong and resilient bones. These recipes cleverly integrate calcium, vitamin D, magnesium, potassium, and other bone-supportive nutrients into delightful and simple-to-make meals.

Let us explore the nourishing world of bone-strengthening recipes, empowering seniors to embrace their golden years with strength and resilience in every step.

1. Salmon Chowder

Ingredients:

- 1 lb salmon fillet, skin removed and cut into chunks
- 2 tablespoons olive oil
- 1 medium onion, chopped
- 2 cloves garlic, minced

- 2 large carrots, peeled and diced
- 2 celery stalks, diced
- Two medium potatoes, peeled and diced
- 4 cups low-sodium chicken or vegetable broth
- 1 cup milk (or dairy-free alternative)
- One cup of corn kernels (fresh, frozen, or canned)
- 1 teaspoon dried thyme
- Salt and pepper to taste
- Fresh parsley for garnish

Instructions:

1. Firstly heat olive oil in a large pot over medium heat. Add chopped onions and minced garlic, sautéing until the onions turn soft and translucent. Incorporate diced carrots, celery, and potatoes, and cook for a few minutes until they slightly soften. Next, pour in low-sodium broth, bringing the mixture to a boil. Reduce the heat and let it simmer for about 15 minutes, ensuring the vegetables become tender.

2. Add salmon chunks, corn kernels, dried thyme, salt, and pepper to the pot. Simmer for an additional 5 minutes or until the salmon is thoroughly cooked. Stir in milk (or a dairy-free alternative) and cook for another 2-3 minutes. Once ready, ladle the nourishing salmon chowder into bowls, garnish with fresh parsley, and serve this delectable and bone-strengthening dish to support the bone health of seniors.

2. Broccoli, Ham, and Cheddar Quiche

Ingredients:

- One prepared pie crust (store-bought or homemade)
- 1 cup chopped cooked ham
- 1 cup steamed broccoli florets

- 1 cup shredded cheddar cheese
- Four large eggs
- 1 cup milk (or dairy-free alternative)
- 1/2 teaspoon dried thyme
- Salt and pepper to taste

Instructions:

1. Start by setting the oven's temperature to 375°F (190°C) and putting the pie dough in a pie dish. Sliced cooked ham, steamed broccoli florets, and shredded cheddar cheese should all be distributed evenly in the pie shell. Whisk the eggs, milk, dried thyme, salt, and pepper in another bowl. Pour the egg mixture over the ham, broccoli, and cheese into the pie shell.

2. For 30-35 minutes, or until the center is set and the crust is golden brown, bake the quiche in the oven. When finished, let the quiche cool a little before cutting and serving.

Enjoy the tasty and calcium-rich broccoli, ham, and cheddar quiche to help maintain the health of your bones.

3. Panna Cotta with Blueberry, Prune Compote, and Cinnamon

Ingredients:

- One cup of heavy cream (or coconut cream for a dairy-free option)
- 1 cup milk (or dairy-free alternative)
- 1/4 cup granulated sugar
- One teaspoon of vanilla extract
- Two teaspoons of unflavored gelatin
- 1/4 cup cold water
- 1 cup blueberries

- 1/2 cup pitted prunes, chopped
- 2 tablespoons honey (or maple syrup)
- 1/2 teaspoon ground cinnamon

Instructions:

1. Pour the heavy cream, milk, sugar, and vanilla essence into a pot and start heating it over medium heat. Turn off the heat after the mixture reaches a simmer.

2. Unflavored gelatin should be combined with cold water in a small dish and allowed to bloom for one minute. The bloomed gelatin must be thoroughly dissolved and stirred into the hot cream mixture.

3. Place the panna cotta mixture into individual serving glasses or molds after that. Panna cotta should be chilled until it hardens, which should take at least 4 hours. Blueberries, prunes that have been chopped, honey (or maple syrup), and cinnamon powder are combined in a different skillet in the meantime. Until the fruits are tender and the compote starts thickening, cook the mixture over medium heat. Before drizzling it over the panna cotta that has been chilled, let the compote cool.

4. Finally, serve this delightful, bone-strengthening panna cotta with blueberry and prune compote. For an elegant touch, garnish with additional blueberries or fresh mint leaves. Indulge in this creamy and nutritious dessert to support your bone health.

4. Veal Cordon Bleu

Ingredients:

- Four veal cutlets (or chicken breasts)
- Four slices of ham
- Four slices of Swiss or Gruyere cheese

- 1/2 cup all-purpose flour
- 2 large eggs, beaten
- 1 cup breadcrumbs
- Salt and pepper to taste
- 2 tablespoons olive oil

Instructions:

1. Set your oven's temperature to 375°F (190°C). After seasoning the veal cutlets with salt and pepper, top each with ham and cheese. If necessary, fasten the veal cutlets with toothpicks before rolling them up.

2. After that, continue by coating the rolled veal cutlets with breadcrumbs, dipping them in beaten eggs, and dredging them in flour. Melt butter in a skillet that can be used in the oven. To obtain a lovely golden brown crust, cook the veal cordon bleu on both sides.

3. Once the crust is golden brown, carefully place the pan in the oven and bake the veal cordon bleu for 15 to 20 minutes, or until the veal is cooked and the cheese has melted.

4. To create a satisfying and bone-strengthening meal, serve this delectable veal cordon bleu with steamed vegetables.

5. Spinach and Ricotta Parcels

Ingredients:

- 1 package phyllo dough
- 2 cups fresh spinach leaves
- 1 cup ricotta cheese
- 1/2 cup shredded mozzarella cheese
- 1/4 cup grated Parmesan cheese
- 1 egg, beaten

- 1 tablespoon olive oil
- Salt and pepper to taste

Instructions:

1. Regulate the oven to 375°F (190°C) and make a baking sheet with parchment paper. Fresh spinach leaves should be sautéed until wilted in olive oil and heated to medium heat in a pan. Add salt and pepper to the dish to enhance the flavor.

2. Following that, combine the sautéed spinach with the ricotta cheese, shredded mozzarella cheese, and grated Parmesan cheese, stirring everything together well. One phyllo sheet should be spread out, and the beaten egg should be delicately brushed. Another piece of phyllo dough should be placed on top, also brushed with beaten egg.

3. Now, cut the double-layered phyllo dough into smaller squares. Spoon a dollop of the spinach and ricotta mixture onto each square, and then fold the squares into parcels, making sure to seal the edges with the beaten egg.

4. After preheating the oven, place the prepared quiche inside and bake it for 30-35 minutes until it sets and the crust turns a delightful golden brown. Once done, allow the quiche to cool briefly before slicing and serving. Embrace the timeless and bone-strengthening Quiche Lorraine, savoring its satisfying and nourishing flavors. It's a meal that everyone can enjoy!

These spinach and ricotta parcels make for a bone-strengthening and scrumptious appetizer or side dish. Serve them to delight your taste buds and support your bone health!

6. Quiche Lorraine

Ingredients:

- 1 prepared pie crust (store-bought or homemade)
- 1 cup diced cooked bacon or ham
- 1 cup shredded Gruyere or Swiss cheese
- Four large eggs
- 1 cup heavy cream (or half-and-half)
- 1/2 teaspoon dried thyme
- Salt and pepper to taste

Instructions:

1. Place the pie dough in a pie dish and regulate the oven to 375°F (190°C). In an even layer, cover the pie crust with chopped cooked bacon or ham and shredded Gruyere or Swiss cheese. Whisk the eggs, heavy cream (or half-and-half), dried thyme, salt, and pepper until well blended in another bowl. Making sure to cover all of the ingredients equally, pour the egg mixture over the bacon and cheese in the pie shell.

2. Put the prepared quiche in the oven and bake it for 30-35 minutes or until it sets and the crust achieves a delightful golden brown hue. After baking, let the quiche cool slightly before slicing and serving.

These bone-strengthening recipes are thoughtfully curated to provide essential nutrients to prevent osteoporosis and promote strong and resilient bones. Incorporating these delicious and nutrient-rich dishes into the diet can empower seniors to take proactive steps towards maintaining bone health and embracing a life of vitality and mobility.

Vitamin D-Packed Foods to Support Bone Density

1: Grilled Salmon with Lemon-Dill Sauce

Ingredients:

- 4 salmon fillets
- 2 tablespoons olive oil
- 1 teaspoon lemon zest
- 2 tablespoons lemon juice
- Two tablespoons fresh dill chopped
- 2 cloves garlic, minced
- Salt and pepper to taste

Instructions:

1. To prepare the salmon, start by preheating the grill to medium-high heat. In a small bowl, create a marinade by mixing olive oil, lemon zest, lemon juice, chopped dill, minced garlic, salt, and pepper. Take the salmon fillets and place them in a shallow dish, pouring the marinade over them. Make sure the fillets are well covered, then cover the dish and place it in the refrigerator to marinate for at least 30 minutes.

2. Once marinated, grill the salmon for approximately 4-5 minutes per side or until it's fully cooked and flakes easily with a fork. Serve the grilled salmon with some lemon slices and a drizzle of the remaining lemon-dill sauce for added flavor.

2: Portobello Mushroom and Spinach Omelette

Ingredients:

- 4 Large eggs
- 1 Cup fresh spinach leaves
- 2 Portobello mushrooms, sliced
- 1/4 cup shredded cheddar cheese
- 2 tablespoons olive oil
- Salt and pepper to taste

Instructions:

1. Firstly, whisk the eggs in a bowl and season them with salt and pepper. After heating the oil, cook the sliced Portobello and mushrooms in a pan until they are soft. Cook the additional fresh spinach leaves until they wilt.

2. Next, pour the whisked eggs over the vegetables and cook the omelet until it sets. On one half of the omelet, sprinkle some shredded cheddar cheese, then fold it over the other half. To get the cheese to melt, give the omelet one more minute to cook.

3. Finally, carefully slide the omelet onto a plate and serve it hot.

This delectable Portobello Mushroom and Spinach Omelette is a nourishing and bone-boosting breakfast or brunch option, rich in vitamin D to support your overall health.

3: Baked Cod with Tomato-Caper Relish

Ingredients:

- Four cod fillets
- 2 tablespoons olive oil
- 1 teaspoon dried oregano
- 1/2 teaspoon garlic powder
- Salt and pepper to taste
- Tomato-Caper Relish:
- 1 cup cherry tomatoes, halved
- 1 tablespoon capers
- 1 tablespoon fresh parsley, chopped
- 1 tablespoon red wine vinegar
- 1 tablespoon extra-virgin olive oil
- Salt and pepper to taste

Instructions:

1. After preheating the oven, place the cod fillets on a baking pan and brush a little olive oil over them. To infuse the fillets with delightful flavors, generously season them with salt, pepper, dried oregano, and garlic powder. Place the cod in the oven and bake for approximately 15 to 18 minutes, or until the fish is fully cooked and easily flakes when tested with a fork. Enjoy this delectable and perfectly seasoned cod straight from the oven!

2. While the cod is baking, you can prepare the delightful tomato-caper relish. In a bowl, combine halved cherry tomatoes, capers, chopped parsley, red wine vinegar, extra-virgin olive oil, salt, and pepper. Toss all the ingredients until they are well mixed and the flavors meld.

3. Once the cod is done, serve it on individual plates and generously top each fillet with a spoonful of the zesty tomato-caper relish.

This recipe offers a delicious and nutritious combination of flavors, making it a delightful meal.

4: Fortified Orange-Carrot Smoothie

Ingredients:

- 2 large oranges, peeled and segmented
- 1 large carrot, peeled and chopped
- A single cup of unsweetened almond milk or any milk variety you prefer.
- 1 tablespoon honey or maple syrup
- 1/2 teaspoon vanilla extract
- Ice cubes (optional)

Instructions:

1. In a blender, combine fresh orange segments, chopped carrots, unsweetened almond milk, honey (or maple syrup), and a splash of vanilla extract. Combine the ingredients and blend until you get a smooth and creamy texture. If you prefer a thicker and colder drink, you can add some ice cubes.

2. Now, pour the revitalizing Orange-Carrot Smoothie into glasses and savor this vitamin D-rich beverage that supports bone density while offering a refreshing and nutritious treat.

5: Greek Yogurt Parfait with Vitamin D-Rich Berries

Ingredients:

- 2 cups Greek yogurt
- 1 cup mixed berries (strawberries, blueberries, raspberries)
- 1/4 cup toasted almond slices
- 2 tablespoons honey
- One teaspoon of grated orange zest

Instructions:

1. Create delightful layers in serving glasses or parfait dishes by alternating Greek yogurt, mixed berries, and toasted almond slices. Drizzle each layer with honey to add a touch of sweetness.

2. Continue layering until the glasses are filled to your desired level of deliciousness. Finish off the parfait by sprinkling grated orange zest on top for a refreshing

and vibrant touch. Enjoy this scrumptious and nutritious treat!

Cognitive function encompasses a spectrum of essential mental abilities like learning, thinking, problem-solving, and decision-making. As we age, cognitive impairment becomes a concern, affecting about two-thirds of seniors around 70. While age remains the primary risk factor, other elements such as family history, education level, brain injury, physical inactivity, and chronic conditions like Parkinson's, heart disease, stroke, and diabetes can also influence cognitive decline.

Intriguingly, our dietary choices play a significant role in shaping cognitive health. The notion of "brain foods" has gained traction as studies reveal how consuming foods impact brain function, memory retention, and overall cognitive well-being. Research suggests that adhering to a low-fat diet may offer protection against cognitive decline, making it a crucial consideration for maintaining cognitive vitality.

In our quest for a sharper mind and sustained cognitive wellness, we present a carefully curated collection of easy-to-prepare healthy recipes. These delightful culinary creations not only tantalize the taste buds but also serve as a proactive investment in better brain health. By incorporating brain-nourishing ingredients into our diets, we take actionable steps toward supporting our cognitive abilities and embracing a fulfilling, cognitively resilient lifestyle.

Omega-3 Fatty Acid Meals for Brain Health

1: Grilled Salmon with Lemon-Dill Sauce

Ingredients:

- Four salmon fillets

- Two tablespoons of olive oil
- One teaspoon of lemon zest
- Two tablespoons of lemon juice
- Two tablespoons fresh dill chopped
- Two cloves garlic, minced
- Salt and pepper to taste

Instructions:

1. Heat the grill to a medium-high temperature to get it ready.

2. Create the marinade by combining olive oil, lemon zest, lemon juice, chopped dill, minced garlic, salt, and pepper in a small bowl.

3. Put the salmon fillets in a dish that isn't too deep. Make sure the fillets are uniformly covered before adding the marinade. The salmon should marinade in the refrigerator for at least 30 minutes, covered in the dish.

4. Grill the marinated salmon for approximately 4-5 minutes per side or until it is thoroughly cooked and flakes easily with a fork.

5. Serve the grilled salmon by garnishing it with extra lemon slices and drizzling the remaining lemon-dill sauce over the top.

2: Walnut and Spinach Salad

Ingredients:

- 4 cups fresh baby spinach leaves
- 1 cup walnuts, toasted and chopped
- 1/2 cup crumbled feta cheese
- 1/4 cup dried cranberries
- Two tablespoons of balsamic vinegar

- One tablespoon honey
- One tablespoon extra-virgin olive oil
- Salt and pepper to taste

Instructions:

1. Combine baby spinach, toasted walnuts, feta cheese crumbles, and dried cranberries in a big salad dish.

2. On a separate, smaller plate, create the dressing by combining balsamic vinegar, honey, extra virgin olive oil, salt, and pepper.

3. Ensure all the ingredients are coated by gently tossing the salad with the dressing drizzled over it.

3: Chia Seed Pudding

Ingredients:

- 1/4 cup chia seeds
- One cup of unsweetened almond milk
- One tablespoon of honey or maple syrup
- 1/2 teaspoon vanilla extract
- Fresh berries for topping

Instructions:

1. In a bowl, thoroughly combine the chia seeds, almond milk without added sugar, honey (or maple syrup), and vanilla essence.

2. Then, to give the chia seeds time to absorb the liquid and thicken, cover the bowl and place it in the refrigerator for at least 4 hours or overnight. Give the mixture one more swirl to produce a smooth consistency before serving.

To enjoy this delicious and nutritious omega-3-packed dessert that promotes brain health and satisfies sweet cravings, top the chia seed pudding with fresh berries.

4: Sardine and Avocado Toast

Ingredients:

- Four slices of whole-grain bread toasted
- One ripe avocado, mashed
- Two cans of sardines in olive oil drained
- One tablespoon of lemon juice
- Fresh cilantro leaves for garnish (optional)
- Salt and pepper to taste

Instructions:

1. Create a creamy spread by mixing mashed avocado together with lemon juice, salt, and pepper in a small bowl.

2. Evenly distribute the avocado spread on the toasted bread slices. Top the avocado spread with sardines, dividing them evenly among the toasts. If desired, garnish with fresh cilantro leaves. Serve immediately for a delicious and satisfying treat.

5: Flaxseed-Crusted Baked Chicken Tenders

Ingredients:

- 1 pound chicken tenders
- 1/2 cup ground flaxseed
- 1/4 cup grated Parmesan cheese
- One teaspoon paprika
- 1/2 teaspoon garlic powder
- 1/2 teaspoon dried thyme

- Salt and pepper to taste
- Two eggs, beaten

Instructions:

1. Start by turning the oven's temperature to 200°C and lining the baking sheet with parchment paper.

2. In a shallow bowl, create the coating mixture by combining ground flaxseed, grated Parmesan cheese, paprika, garlic powder, dried thyme, salt, and pepper.

3. Each chicken tender should be completely covered in the beaten eggs before dipping into the flaxseed mixture.

4. Place the chicken tenders that have been coated on the prepared baking sheet.

5. When the chicken is thoroughly cooked, and the coating is golden and crispy, bake the chicken for 20 to 25 minutes.

The omega-3-rich flaxseed coating adds a brain-boosting twist to traditional baked chicken tenders.

Antioxidant-Rich Snacks to Enhance Memory

1: Berry Blast Smoothie

Ingredients:

- 1 cup mixed berries (blueberries, strawberries, raspberries)
- 1/2 cup Greek yoghurt
- 1/2 cup almond milk
- One tablespoon of chia seeds

- One tablespoon honey
- 1/2 teaspoon vanilla extract
- A handful of spinach leaves (optional)

Instructions:

1. Blend all the ingredients til the sauce is smooth and creamy. Add extra almond milk as necessary if you like a thinner consistency.

2. Once ready, pour the smoothie into a glass and savour its refreshing taste and memory-enhancing benefits, thanks to its antioxidant-rich ingredients.

This delightful smoothie is not only delicious but also supports your cognitive health. Enjoy!

2: Quinoa Salad with Pomegranate and Walnuts

Ingredients:

- 1 cup cooked quinoa
- 1/2 cup pomegranate arils
- 1/4 cup chopped walnuts
- 1/4 cup chopped fresh parsley
- Two tablespoons extra-virgin olive oil
- One tablespoon of lemon juice
- One teaspoon honey
- Salt and pepper to taste

Instructions:

1. Using a large bowl, mix the cooked quinoa, pomegranate arils, chopped walnuts, and fresh parsley.

2. Mix the dressing ingredients—extra virgin olive oil, lemon juice, honey, salt, and pepper—in a separate small bowl.

3. Toss the quinoa mixture lightly to evenly distribute the dressing over all ingredients. In addition to being delicious and nutrient-rich, this quinoa salad has memory-enhancing properties.

3: Roasted Turmeric Cauliflower

Ingredients:

- 1 medium cauliflower, cut into florets
- 2 tablespoons of olive oil
- 1 teaspoon of ground turmeric
- 1/2 teaspoon ground cumin
- 1/2 teaspoon ground coriander
- 1/4 teaspoon garlic powder
- Salt and pepper to taste

Instructions:

1. First, set the oven's temperature to 425°F (220°C). Cauliflower florets should be mixed with olive oil, salt, pepper, garlic powder, powdered cumin, ground turmeric, and ground coriander in a large bowl. Stir the mixture until the oil and spices are applied equally to the cauliflower.

2. Next, spread the seasoned cauliflower on a baking sheet in a single layer. Roast it in the oven for 20-25 minutes or until the cauliflower becomes tender and develops a delightful golden brown color.

4: Green Tea Poached Salmon

Ingredients:

- Four salmon fillets
- 3 cups brewed green tea, cooled
- Two tablespoons of low-sodium soy sauce
- Two cloves garlic, minced
- 1-inch piece of fresh ginger, sliced
- One tablespoon honey
- One teaspoon of sesame oil
- 1/4 teaspoon red pepper flakes (optional)
- Sliced green onions for garnish

Instructions:

1. In a large skillet or shallow pan, create the poaching liquid by combining brewed green tea, low-sodium soy sauce, minced garlic, sliced ginger, honey, sesame oil, and red pepper flakes (if desired). Take the mixture to a simmer over medium heat.

2. Once the poaching liquid is ready, add the salmon fillets to the skillet, ensuring they are fully submerged. Allow the salmon to poach in the liquid for 8-10 minutes or until thoroughly cooked.

3. Carefully remove the poached salmon from the liquid and place it on serving plates. For an added touch, garnish with sliced green onions.

This delicious and flavorful poached salmon makes for an impressive and healthy dish that will surely be enjoyed by everyone at the table!

5: Dark Chocolate Avocado Mousse

Ingredients:

- Two ripe avocados

- ¼ cup unsweetened cocoa powder
- ¼ cup of pure maple syrup or honey
- ¼ cup almond milk
- One teaspoon of vanilla extract
- 1 pinch of salt
- Fresh berries for topping (optional)

Instructions:

1. In a food processor, blend ripe avocados, unsweetened cocoa powder, pure maple syrup (or honey), almond, as well as milk, vanilla extract, and a pinch of salt until the mixture becomes smooth and creamy. Taste the mousse and adjust the sweetness to your liking.

2. Pour the mousse made with dark chocolate and avocado into individual glasses or serving bowls. The mousse should be chilled in the fridge for at least 30 minutes before serving for the greatest texture and flavor.

3. To enhance the dessert with antioxidants and a delightful touch, top each serving with fresh berries.

Brain-Healthy Desserts for a Sweet Treat

1: Blueberry-Almond Oatmeal Cookies

Ingredients:

- 1 cup rolled oats
- ½ cup almond flour
- ½ cup whole wheat flour
- ½ teaspoon baking soda
- ¼ teaspoon salt
- ¼ cup of coconut oil

- ¼ cup of pure maple syrup or honey
- 1 large egg
- 1 teaspoon of vanilla extract
- ½ cup fresh blueberries

Instructions:

1. Mix the rolled oats, whole wheat flour, baking soda, and salt in a mixing dish. In another dish, mix the melted coconut oil, honey, egg, maple syrup, and vanilla extract.

2. As you gradually incorporate the wet ingredients into the dry ones, whisk everything together well. Fold in the fresh blueberries gently. As usual, preheat the oven, and prepare a parchment-lined baking sheet.

3. Scoop tablespoon-sized portions of the cookie dough onto the lined baking sheet, ensuring they are spaced apart. Slightly flatten each cookie using the back of a spoon. Bake for 10-12 minutes or until the edges turn golden brown. Prior to moving the cookies to a wire rack to finish cooling, let them cool on the baking sheet for a short while.

2: Dark Chocolate Avocado Truffles

Ingredients:

- 2 ripe avocados

- ½ cup dark cocoa powder

- ¼ cup of pure maple syrup or honey

- 1 teaspoon of vanilla extract

- 1 pinch of salt

- ¼ cup unsweetened cocoa powder or shredded coconut for coating

Instructions:

1. In a food processor, combine ripe avocados, dark chocolate powder, pure maple syrup (or honey), vanilla essence, and a sprinkle of salt until the mixture is smooth and creamy. Refrigerate the mixture for about 30 minutes to allow it to firm up.

2. Once chilled, take small portions of the mixture and shape them into truffle balls. Coat each truffle with either unsweetened cocoa powder or shredded coconut. Place the coated truffles on a plate or tray and refrigerate for 15-20 minutes before serving.

These delightful dark chocolate avocado truffles are not only guilt-free but also nourishing for your brain while satisfying your sweet cravings.

3: Greek Yogurt and Mixed Berries Parfait

Ingredients:

- 1 cup Greek yoghurt
- 1 cup mixed berries (blueberries, strawberries, raspberries)
- 2 tablespoons honey
- ¼ cup granola
- Fresh mint leaves for garnish (optional)

Instructions:

1. For a brain-healthy treat, assemble this delightful yoghurt and mixed berries parfait in a glass or parfait dish. Begin by layering Greek yoghurt and mixed berries and drizzling honey over each layer.

2. Layer the ingredients until the glass is filled to your preference. Complete the parfait by generously sprinkling granola and adding fresh mint leaves as a garnish if desired.

This refreshing dessert or wholesome breakfast option is sure to please and nourish your body and mind. Enjoy the goodness of yoghurt and mixed berries as a tasty and beneficial addition to your day!

4: Chia Seed Pudding with Mango

Ingredients:

- 1/4 cup chia seeds
- 1 cup unsweetened almond milk (or any milk of your choice)
- 1 tablespoon honey or maple syrup
- 1/2 teaspoon vanilla extract
- 1 ripe mango, diced
- Toasted coconut flakes for topping (optional)

Instructions:

1. Mix the chia seeds, unsweetened almond milk, honey (or maple syrup), and vanilla extract well in a bowl. Give the mixture time to rest for the chia seeds to absorb the liquid. Give it one more stir, then chill for at least four hours or overnight to get a thicker consistency.

2. Once the chia seed pudding has been set, spoon it into serving bowls or glasses. Add diced mango and toasted coconut flakes to enhance the texture and flavour.

This refreshing chia seed pudding with mango not only offers a satisfying dessert option but also provides a brain-boosting treat to enjoy guilt-free.

5: Walnut and Banana Muffins

Ingredients:

- 1 cup whole wheat flour
- 1/2 cup almond flour
- 1 teaspoon of baking powder
- 1/2 teaspoon baking soda
- 1/4 teaspoon salt
- 2 ripe bananas, mashed
- ¼ cup of coconut oil melted
- ¼ cup of pure maple syrup or honey
- 1 large egg
- 1 teaspoon of vanilla extract
- ½ cup chopped walnuts

Instructions:

1. After that, prepare a muffin tray by lining it with paper liners and heat the oven to 350°F (175°C). Combine salt, baking soda, baking powder, whole wheat flour, and almond flour in a large basin. Combine the bananas, melted coconut oil, honey or pure maple syrup, egg, and vanilla essence in a separate dish.

2. Mix until mixed after gradually incorporating the wet components into the dry ones. Add the chopped walnuts and combine. Fill each cup in the hot muffin tray about two-thirds full by scooping the batter into them.

3. Until a toothpick put into the center of one of the muffins comes out clean, bake the muffins for 18 to 20 minutes.

4. After the muffins have finished cooling in the pan for a few minutes, move them to a wire rack to finish cooling.

These mouthwatering dishes provide a lovely fusion of flavors and necessary nutrients for the wellness of your brain.

SECTION FIVE: PHYSICAL ACTIVITIES AND WELLNESS TIPS FOR ACTIVE SENIORS

Age is a number, and for adults aged 65 and older, staying physically active holds the key to a strong and fulfilling life. As the years gracefully advance, a well-rounded mix of aerobic, muscle-strengthening, and balance activities becomes the secret elixir to keep bodies resilient and agile. Regular physical activity fosters independence and enriches the quality of life while effectively warding off chronic illnesses.

In this journey towards vitality, it's comforting to know that it's never too late to embark on a path of physical activity. The key lies in selecting activities that match your abilities and ignite the joy within you. By indulging in activities that bring happiness and align with your capabilities, you forge a lasting bond with fitness, ensuring a steadfast commitment to a healthier and more vibrant you. So, let's lace up those sneakers and uncover the wonders that await as we venture into active ageing.

Low-Impact Exercises for Joint Health

Low-impact exercises are ideal for seniors as they are gentle on the joints while providing effective workouts. Walking is one of the simplest yet most effective low-impact exercises seniors can incorporate into their routines. It promotes cardiovascular health, strengthens leg muscles, and can be enjoyed indoors and outdoors. Swimming and water aerobics are great options for maintaining joint health since the buoyancy of the water eases pressure on the joints and provides resistance for muscle building.

Balance and Flexibility Exercises for Fall Prevention

Balance and flexibility exercises are essential for fall prevention and maintaining mobility. Yoga and Tai Chi are popular among seniors, as they improve balance and flexibility and promote relaxation and stress reduction. These exercises focus on slow, controlled movements that help seniors develop better balance and coordination, reducing the risk of falls and related injuries.

Strength Training to Maintain Muscle Mass

Strength training is crucial for seniors to combat age-related muscle loss and maintain strength. Resistance exercises using light weights, resistance bands, or body weight can effectively build muscle mass and bone density. Strength training also enhances joint stability and increases overall physical independence. Exercises must be performed with proper form and under the guidance of a trained fitness teacher in order to ensure their safety and effectiveness.

Creating an Active Lifestyle in Daily Routines

Fostering an active lifestyle that supports long-term health and well-being requires incorporating physical exercise into everyday activities.

Incorporating Physical Activity into Daily Tasks

Simple adjustments to daily tasks can effortlessly infuse physical activity into a senior's routine. Taking the stairs instead of the elevator, parking the car farther away to walk a little extra, and doing household chores actively, such as vacuuming or gardening, contribute to increased daily activity levels.

Outdoor Activities for Enjoyable Workouts

Engaging in outdoor activities promotes physical health, provides a refreshing change of scenery, and boosts mood.

Seniors can consider activities like brisk walking in the park, cycling on dedicated trails, or exploring nature with hiking groups. These activities offer the dual benefit of exercise and connecting with nature, which has positively affected mental well-being.

Group Activities and Social Engagement for Motivation

Participating in group activities encourages physical activity and provides a social support system, reducing feelings of isolation. Many communities offer senior exercise classes, dance classes, or sports clubs where seniors can interact with peers while staying active. The camaraderie and shared motivation within these groups often lead to better adherence to an active lifestyle.

For elders to preserve their health, independence, and overall well-being, regular physical exercise is crucial. Low-impact activities safeguard joint health, improve balance and flexibility, lower the chance of falling, and strength training maintains muscle mass.

Integrating physical activity into daily tasks, enjoying outdoor workouts, and engaging in group activities foster an active lifestyle that enhances the quality of life for active seniors. By staying proactive about physical activity, seniors can embrace the joys of an active and vibrant life throughout their golden years.

CONCLUSION

In the grand tapestry of life, the chapter of active ageing unfolds with grace and determination. As we reach the golden years, the stars of nutrition and physical activity align to guide us towards vitality and well-being. Like a harmonious melody, a balanced diet orchestrates a cascade of benefits for active seniors. The power of nourishment is their key to unlocking a treasure trove of energy, supporting bone health, and fortifying their bodies with essential vitamins and minerals. As the colors of a rainbow weave through the skies, the diverse palette of nutrients paints a masterpiece of immunity, shielding seniors from the grasp of illness and infusing their lives with vigor.

Amidst this symphony, physical activity takes up its baton, leading seniors in an enchanting dance of movement. The stages set by low-impact exercises reveal the secrets to joint health, bestowing strength and agility with each step taken. As they glide through the waters of swimming and water aerobics, the buoyant embrace nurtures their bodies while the resistance molds their muscles into works of art. In the gentle cadence of walking, seniors find solace as it enriches their hearts with the rhythm of life, keeping them agile and independent.

As the stars align, the path of active ageing illuminates the way to overall well-being and a life of unparalleled quality. Like a constellation of blessings, these lifestyle choices enrich mental clarity, promote sound sleep, and elevate mood, culminating in a harmonious existence. With spirits alight, active seniors embark on a journey filled with laughter, friendship, and joy, for they understand that age is never a barrier to a fulfilling life.

In this guide, we extend our hands, offering encouragement and support to every senior on this magical journey. Let the radiant light of nutrition and physical activity be your guiding stars, leading you to a life filled with vibrancy and fulfilment. Together, we shall paint a world where active ageing shines like the sun, illuminating future generations' lives. May you, dear seniors, forever be the embodiments of ageless wisdom and the champions of living life to its fullest.